# THE COMPLETE 2024 LOW FIBER DIET COOKBOOK

**Delicious and Tasty Low Residue Recipes to Improve your Digestive System with 7 Days Meal Plan for Other Similar Diseases**

*LUCKY WILSON*

# *CITATION IN VIEW..*

# Table of Contents

# INTRODUCTION

A low fiber diet, or low residue diet, limits the amount of fiber you eat each day. "Residue" refers to food that ends up in your gastrointestinal (GI) tract or stool because your body cannot digest it. Often, these are high fiber foods.

A low fiber diet aims to give your digestive system a rest by:
• reducing the amount of undigested food moving through the gut
• easing the amount of work the digestive system is doing
• reducing the amount of stool produced
• easing abdominal pain, diarrhea, and other symptoms

Low residue diets have been removed from the American Academy of Nutrition and Dietetics' Nutrition Care Manual. However, the authors of a 2015 review suggest that low fiber diets may still have several benefits. For example, a healthcare professional may recommend following a low fiber diet if you're living with a GI condition or if you're preparing for surgery, such as a colonoscopy. It's important to note that low fiber diets are not intended for weight loss. Without proper guidance, the diet can cause unintended side effects and make symptoms worse in the long run.

## Types of fiber

Dietary fiber plays a role in stool formation, density, and acceleration. It's typically divided into two types:
• Soluble fiber absorbs water during digestion and turns into a soft, gel-like substance. This type of fiber is less likely to irritate your GI tract. However, it may still increase symptoms like gas and bloating because soluble fiber-rich foods contain prebiotics that feed gut bacteria.
• Insoluble fiber doesn't dissolve in the stomach. It's found in many foods not recommended to eat during a low fiber diet because the undigested fragments may irritate the gut.

## Tips for a low fiber diet

Before starting a low fiber diet, speak with a healthcare professional. They can offer advice on foods to eat and avoid, as well as help determine the proper amount of fiber for you to eat.
Some tips to help you manage your fiber intake include:
• Buying foods with less than 2 g of fiber per serving
• Peeling your vegetables and fruits
• Avoiding foods that may trigger symptoms
• Staying hydrated to help avoid constipation
• Avoiding insoluble fibers
It might also help to meet with a dietitian to get specific meal plans and guidance on eating a low fiber diet.

# Meal plan for Low Fiber Diet

Here are examples of meals you can eat on a low fiber diet:
Breakfast
• Hard-boiled eggs with buttered white toast and unsweetened vegetable juice
• Low fiber breakfast cereals, such as cornflakes, puffed rice, and porridge
Lunch
• Tuna sandwich with an unseeded white roll and mayonnaise
• White rice with a chicken breast
Dinner
• Lightly-seasoned salmon with mashed potatoes
• An omelet with roasted sweet potatoes

# What are the benefits of a low fiber diet?

A low fiber diet can help give your digestive system a break because fiber takes more effort for your body to digest.
Your doctor might recommend trying this diet for a short time if you have one of the following:
• irritable bowel syndrome (IBS)
• Crohn's disease
• ulcerative colitis
• diverticulitis

- Diarrhea
- Abdominal cramps
- Irritation or damage in the digestive tract
- Bowel narrowing caused by a tumor
- Recovery from GI surgery, including colostomy and ileostomy
- Current radiation therapy or other treatments that might affect the GI tract

## What To Eat On A Low-Fiber Diet

While there is currently no standard recommendation on how much you need to limit your fiber, some experts suggest eating less than 10–15 grams of fiber per day.

Along with avoiding high-fiber foods, recommendations include avoiding spicy and highly processed foods, such as deli meats, hot dogs, sausage, and deep-fried foods, as these foods can be tough on digestion.

Vegetables

- Lettuce (shredded and in small quantities), peeled cucumbers without seeds, zucchini, yellow squash without seeds, spinach, pumpkin, eggplant, skinless potatoes, green beans, wax beans, asparagus, beets, and carrots.

Fruits

- Fruit juices without pulp, many canned fruits, and fruit sauces.

• Very ripe: apricots, bananas, cantaloupe, honeydew melon, watermelon, nectarines, papayas, peaches, and plums.

Breads and grains

• White breads, dry cereals, white pasta, and crackers.

• Make sure these foods have less than 2 grams of fiber per serving.

Protein

• Cooked meat, fish, poultry, eggs, smooth peanut butter, and tofu.

• Make sure meat is tender and soft, and not chewy.

Oils

• Butter, margarine, oils, mayonnaise, whipped cream, and smooth sauces and dressings.

• Smooth condiments.

Dairy

• Yogurt, kefir, cottage cheese, milk, pudding, creamy soup, or hard cheese

• Angel food cake, animal crackers, custard, gelatin, ginger snaps, graham crackers, saltine crackers, sherbet, sorbet, vanilla wafers, yogurt (plain or vanilla).

## How do I start eating fiber again

Reducing your intake of fiber may help improve symptoms in the short term. However, it's important to gradually reintroduce fiber into your diet when these symptoms improve.

The authors of a 2022 review suggest that a high fiber diet may have several benefits for people living with irritable bowel disease (IBD). These may include:

• decreasing inflammation
• improving immune response and overall health
• restoring gut microbiome
• reducing the risk of colorectal cancer

You can start by adding a small portion of one high fiber food per day. If this doesn't cause any symptoms, you can then add it back into your diet.

The amount of fiber you need depends on several factors, such as age, sex, and underlying health conditions.


## Frequently asked questions

What foods are low in fiber for a colonoscopy?

A healthcare professional may recommend eating low fiber foods before getting a colonoscopy. These may include:
• refined carbohydrates, such as white bread, pasta, and rice
• some boiled or steamed vegetables
• some fruit and vegetable juices
• lean protein sources, such as eggs, chicken, and tofu

# Can you eat oatmeal on a low fiber diet?

Oats are mostly high in soluble fiber. According to the American Cancer Society, this type of fiber is less likely to irritate your intestines as much as insoluble fiber. However, it's best to eat a small portion of oatmeal and see how you feel afterward. If it triggers any symptoms, stay away from oatmeal.

## What is a low fiber diet for breakfast?

Some low fiber breakfast foods include:
• eggs
• white toast
• some breakfast cereals, such as cornflakes and puffed rice
• some fruits

Takeaway

A low fiber diet may help you manage symptoms if you're living with a health condition that affects your digestive system.

However, it's important to only follow a low fiber diet under the guidance of a healthcare professional. They can help you determine the best diet plan for you.

# What Foods Are Easy to Digest?

What are the easiest and fastest foods to digest?
Foods low in fiber are typically easy to digest. These can include:
• canned or cooked fruit without seeds or skin
• canned or cooked vegetables without seeds or skin
• lean meat and other lean protein
• refined grains, like white bread
• low fat dairy products, if you aren't lactose intolerant
• fermented foods, like sauerkraut and pickles

## Canned or cooked fruits without the skin or seeds

Whole fruits contain high amounts of fiber, but cooking them helps break down the fiber significantly, which makes them easier to digest. Peeling the skin and removing any seeds helps lower the amount of fiber.
Low fiber fruits include:
• Very ripe banana
• Cantaloupe
• Honeydew melon
• Watermelon
• Avocado
• Applesauce

## Canned or cooked vegetables without the skin or seeds

Just like fruit, whole vegetables have a lot of fiber. Once cooked, the fiber is partially broken down and easier to digest. You can cook your vegetables at home or find canned varieties at your local grocery store.
Low fiber vegetables include peeled and well-cooked:
• Potatoes
• Yellow squash
• Spinach
• Pumpkin
• Beets
• Green beans
• Carrots

## Lean meats and other sources of protein

People tend to digest main courses of lean protein well. This can include:
• Chicken
• Turkey
• Fish
• Tender cuts of beef or pork and ground meats
• Eggs
• Creamy nut butter
• Tofu

How you prepare meat can also affect how easy it is to digest. Instead of frying it, try grilling, broiling, baking, or poaching it.

High fat can sometimes be uncomfortable to digest because fat moves through the gut more slowly, so you may want to consider removing poultry skin and draining fat from cooked ground meats.

Refined grains

Refined flours (grains) have been modified to remove the bran and germ, making them easier to digest. Common examples include:
• White bread
• Plain bagels
• Pasta noodles
• Pretzels
• White crackers

You can also find low fiber dry or cooked cereals at the grocery store.

Dairy products

If you're lactose intolerant, dairy may upset your digestion or cause diarrhea. Look for products that are lactose-free or low in lactose.

Otherwise, low fat dairy is low in fiber and may be easy to digest for many people. Dairy products to try can include:

• Low fat plain milk
• Low fat cheese
• Low fat yogurt
• Low fat cottage cheese

Fermented foods

While not low in fiber, fermented foods have the potential to help digestion. Fermented foods can include:
• Sauerkraut
• Kimchi
• Pickles
• Other pickled vegetables
These foods typically contain "friendly" bacteria like probiotics, which support gut health. Probiotics can also produce digestive enzymes that predigest food and help you better absorb nutrients.

## Foods that typically aren't easy to digest

Some foods contain lots of fiber and can be harder to digest.

Fresh or dried fruits
Most fresh fruits contain a hefty amount of fiber, especially if they have skins or seeds. You may want to avoid the following varieties in particular:

• Berries

• Coconut

• Canned fruit cocktail

• Pineapple

You may need to avoid any fruit juices that contain pulp. Citrus fruits may be especially difficult for people with gastroesophageal reflux disease (GERD).

Raw vegetables

You may need to avoid raw vegetables as they contain much more intact fiber than cooked or canned options.

High fiber raw vegetables you may need to avoid include:

• Beans

• Broccoli

• Brussels sprouts

• Cabbage

• Cauliflower

• Corn

• Mushrooms

• Onion

• Peas

• Peppers

• Tomatoes

Tough meats and other protein sources

Any meats that are tough or fibrous may be hard to digest. These include:

• Meats with casings, such as hot dogs, sausage, and kielbasa

• Lunch meats
• Shellfish

Other protein sources may give you some trouble going through your digestive system. These can include:

• Beans and legumes
• Chunky peanut butter
• Whole nuts
• Whole seeds

Whole grains

Whole-grain bread, pastries, and other whole-grain flour-based items may be more difficult to digest. You may need to avoid grain products, like crackers and cereals, that contain certain ingredients, such as:

• Raisins or other dried fruits
• Nuts
• Seeds
• Bran

Other foods

People who are lactose intolerant may want to avoid most dairy products.

Generally speaking, other foods and drinks that may be difficult to digest can include:

• high fat foods like butter, oils, and full-fat dairy products
• alcohol
• carbonated drinks like soda
• caffeinated drinks like coffee
• fresh or whole spices

• Jams and jellies that contain seeds
• Spicy or fried foods

## What to Eat After Colonoscopy

A colonoscopy is a screening test, generally done under conscious sedation provided by a nurse or deep sedation provided by an anesthesiologist. It's used to detect potential health problems in the colon, such as polyps and colorectal cancer.

What you eat and drink after the procedure is important. The preparations you went through to prepare for the colonoscopy are dehydrating, so putting fluids and electrolytes back into your system is vital. For the rest of that day and the day after, you'll be advised to drink lots of fluid and to eat soft, easily digestible foods which won't irritate your colon.

These dietary safeguards are typically required for one day only, but everyone is different. If your system can't tolerate your usual diet immediately, continue to eat soft and liquid-based foods for an extra day or two.

# What is the best meal after a colonoscopy?

After a colonoscopy, you'll eat and drink things that are gentle on your digestive system. Drinking lots of fluid and fluid-based foods will help you avoid dehydration.
In most cases, you would be sedated for the procedure, which is another reason why it may be better to start off with clear liquids or soup.

Other foods you can eat after a colonoscopy

Your doctor may then recommend you follow a soft, low-residue diet. This consists of a limited amount of dairy plus low fiber foods, which are easy to digest and produce less stool.
Foods and drinks to have the day after your colonoscopy include:
• Drinks with electrolytes
• Water
• Fruit juice
• Vegetable juice
• Herbal tea
• Saltine crackers
• Graham crackers
• Soup
• Applesauce
• Scrambled eggs
• Tender, cooked vegetables

- Canned fruit, such as peaches
- Yogurt
- Jell-O
- Popsicles
- Pudding
- Mashed or baked potato
- White bread or toast
- Smooth nut butter
- Soft white fish
- Apple butter

## What not to eat after a colonoscopy

A colonoscopy only takes around 30 minutes, but your system may still need recuperation time. This is partly due to the procedure itself and partly due to the bowel prep, you went through before it.

To aid healing, avoiding foods that are hard to digest the day after is beneficial. This includes anything that might irritate your bowels, such as spicy foods and those high in fiber. Heavy, greasy foods may also increase feelings of nausea after general anesthesia.

Air is introduced into the colon during the procedure so that it can remain open. Because of this, you may expel more gas afterward than you normally do. If so, you may wish to avoid carbonated beverages, which add more gas to your system. If you had a polyp removed, your doctor may recommend additional dietary guidelines. These include avoiding foods, such as seeds, nuts, and popcorn, for an additional two weeks.

Foods and drinks to avoid the day after your colonoscopy include:
• Alcoholic beverages
• Steak, or any tough, hard-to-digest meat
• Whole grain bread
• Whole grain crackers or crackers with seeds
• Raw vegetables
• Corn
• Legumes
• Brown rice
• Fruit with the skin on
• Dried fruit, such as raisins
• Coconut
• Spices, such as garlic, curry, and red pepper
• Highly seasoned foods
• Crunchy nut butter
• Popcorn
• Fried food
• Nuts

# Best practices for taking care of your colon

Your colon-which is also known as the large intestine or bowels-is a vital part of the digestive system.
Taking care of your colon requires more than just regular screenings. It also means eating healthy, keeping your body mass index in a healthy range, and avoiding unhealthy lifestyle choices.

About 10-30% of people with colon cancer have family members with the disease, suggesting a genetic component. That said, healthy habits also have a large effect on your colon health. An older 2015 study reported obesity-especially abdominal obesity-and type 2 diabetes are risk factors for colon cancer. A newer 2019 study showed that undergoing bariatric surgery can also reduce the chance of getting several cancers, including colon cancer, by 33%. Dietary factors are cited within the article as increasing this risk.

Healthy foods to eat include:
• Fruits
• Vegetables
• Lean protein
• Whole grains
• Low fat dairy, such as yogurt and skim milk
Unhealthy foods to avoid include:
• Desserts and high-sugar foods

• Foods high in saturated fat, such as fast food

• Red meat

• Processed meat

Smoking cigarettes, or using other tobacco products, isn't advisable for good colon health.

Staying active-especially by exercising-is also important for your colon health. Exercise helps reduce insulin levels. It also helps keep weight down.

## Frequently asked questions

How long after a colonoscopy can you eat normally?
You can resume eating right after a colonoscopy, but it's a good idea to introduce food slowly and begin with liquid foods.

What should I eat to restore my gut after a colonoscopy?
Research shows that 20% of people can experience uncomfortable abdominal symptoms after a colonoscopy, which may be related to a disrupted gut microbiome. Taking probiotics may help you restore your gut microbiome after a colonoscopy.

What is the fastest way to recover from a colonoscopy?
Most people recover quickly from a colonoscopy, but it's important to follow all your doctor's instructions. These may include avoiding any strenuous activity and taking a

day off work before returning to your normal routine. If you experience any unusual symptoms, tell your doctor right away.


Takeaway

A colonoscopy can detect problems in your colon, such as polyps or cancer. The preparation for it is dehydrating, so drinking a lot of fluid after the procedure is important.

What you eat and drink after this procedure is also very important. Your doctor may recommend a restricted diet, such as just soft foods that require little digestion. if you follow your doctor's instructions, you should recover and resume eating normally within a day.

# Low Fiber Diet Recipes

Low fodmap pasta with salmon and spinach

* Total Time: 20 mins
* Servings: 2
* Diet: Gluten Free

INGREDIENTS
* 150 g (5.3 oz) gluten-free spaghetti
* 250 g (8.8 oz) fresh spinach
* 250 g (8.8 oz) canned mushrooms or oyster mushrooms
* 125 g (4.4 oz) lactose-free cream cheese
* 150 g (5.3 oz) smoked salmon
* Lemon juice
* 1/2 tsp pepper
* 1/2 tsp salt
* Optional: a small handful of parsley, the green part of leek or spring onion for garnish

INSTRUCTIONS
* Bring a pan with water to boil and cook the spaghetti according to the instructions on the package.
* Heat some olive oil in a pan.
* If you use fresh salmon, you can cut the salmon into small pieces and fry it for a few minutes on low / medium heat.
* Add the spinach and fry for a few minutes.

• Drain the mushrooms and rinse them well. Add them to the spinach and heat for a few minutes.
• If you use oyster mushrooms, scrub them clean and cut them into small pieces. Add them to the pan and fry for a few minutes.
• Put the cream cheese into a bowl and season with a splash of lemon juice, pepper, salt and optionally some fresh parsley.
• Add the cream cheese to the pan and heat for a few minutes, while you stir now and then.
• If you use smoked salmon: cut the salmon into small pieces and add to the pan. Heat the sauce through for a few minutes.
• Taste and season with extra salt, pepper or lemon juice if necessary.
• Drain the spaghetti and divide over two plates. Scoop the sauce on top. Garnish with some fresh parsley and optionally the green parts of spring onion or leek, cut into rings.


Healthy Fried Rice

Prep Time: 10 minutes
Cook Time: 30 minutes
Total Time: 40 minutes

Ingredients
• 1 tablespoon olive oil

• 1 lb ButcherBox Boneless Skinless Chicken Breasts cut into 1 inch cubes
• 1 cup onion finely chopped (1 medium onion)
• 1 tablespoon garlic finely minced
• 1 cup red bell pepper diced in small squares (1 large pepper)
• 1 cup carrots peeled then finely chopped
• 2 eggs
• 1/4 teaspoon pepper
• 1/4 teaspoon ground ginger
• 1/4 teaspoon red pepper flakes optional- omit if you like less spice
• 1 tablespoon toasted sesame oil
• 1/2 cup coconut aminos
• 1 cup frozen green peas thawed
• 2 cups cooked white or brown rice (about 2/3 dry brown rice)

Instructions
• Cook rice according to the directions. Rice cooking time will vary depending on what type/method you use.
• In a pan, heat 1/2 tablespoon olive oil. Sauté chicken for 15-20 minutes until brown on edges. Remove chicken from the pan and set aside.
• In the same pan, add additional 1/2 tablespoon of olive oil. Heat the oil and sauté onions and garlic for 5 minutes.
• After 5 minutes add in peppers and carrots. Sauté for an additional 5 minutes until they start to soften.
• Push the veggie mixture to one side of the pan.

• In a small bowl, whisk together eggs until combined. Add eggs to the pan and scramble on the empty side of the pan.
• Once eggs are cooked (about 1-2 minutes), stir together with veggie mixture.
• Add pepper, ginger, red pepper flakes, toasted sesame oil, coconut aminos, thawed peas, cooked rice and cooked chicken back to the pot. Stir over low heat until combined and warm.
• Serve with sesame seeds or chopped scallions + enjoy.


Healthy Fried Rice Recipe

• Prep Time: 5 mins
• Cook Time: 10 mins
• Total Time: 15 mins
• Yield: 2–4 servings
• Category: Main Dish
• Method: Saute Cuisine: Asian

Ingredients
• 1 tablespoon avocado oil (or other healthy cooking oil), divided
• 3 large eggs
• 5–6 scallions (aka green onions), root and 2 inches of green top removed, chopped (about 1/2 cup)
• 1 large carrot, shredded or julienned (about 1/2 cup)
• 1/2 cup frozen peas
• 2 cups cooked brown rice

• 3 tablespoons organic tamari or low sodium soy sauce
• 1 teaspoon rice vinegar (no sugar added)
• 1 teaspoon toasted sesame oil
• 1/2 teaspoon freshly grated ginger
• Big pinch of sea salt (more or less to taste)
• A few spins freshly ground black pepper

Instructions
1. Heat 1/2 tablespoon oil over medium heat.
2. In a mixing bowl, whisk the eggs into a uniform mixture until well combine and season with a small pinch of sea salt and fresh black pepper.
3. Add the eggs to the pan and scramble. Once cooked remove the scrambled eggs from the pan to a plate and reserve for later.
4. Add the remaining 1/2 tablespoon oil to the pan over medium heat; add the scallions and carrot and sauté 3-4 minutes until softened.
5. Add the frozen peas to the pan, then add the rice, tamari, rice vinegar, toasted sesame oil and ginger. Stir well to combine, the heat from the pan will quickly defrost the peas.
6. Turn off the heat and stir in the scrambled eggs. Season with a pinch of sea salt if needed–it will depend on the sodium content of the tamari and other ingredients.
7. Turn the heat to low and cook another 5 minutes until the entire dish is warmed through.

8. Water chestnuts, bean sprouts, edamame, just about any other veggie you like, or plain shredded chicken would also be a delicious addition to this dish.

Notes

1. Grab some cooked brown rice on the hot bar at the store to make this even easier. Frozen brown rice also works, defrost it first. Or, cook your rice from scratch according to the package instructions. Any white rice can also be substituted if you prefer.
2. Tamari is gluten-free soy sauce and tastes just like regular soy sauce. You can find it in the ethnic aisle of most grocery stores or at an Asian market. Substitute low-sodium soy sauce if desired.

## LOW FAT CRISPY POTATOES

Yield: 4
Prep Time: 10 minutes
Cook Time: 40 minutes
Total Time: 50 minutes
Crispy new potatoes, par-boiled and roasted until crisp with herbs, seasoning and no oil.

## INGREDIENTS
- 1 kg / 2.2 lbs baby potatoes
- (optional) Low-cal olive oil spray
- 2 tsp garlic powder

- 1 tsp onion powder
- 1 tbsp dried mixed herbs
- Salt and pepper, to taste
- Fresh parsley, to serve

## INSTRUCTIONS

1. Preheat the oven to 200c / 390f and line a large roasting tin with parchment paper or a silicone baking mat. Alternatively, spray with 1 cal olive oil spray.
2. Rinse the potatoes then cut them in half, at an angle, to create as much flat surface as possible for optimum crispiness. Leave small potatoes whole and cut the larger ones into thirds or quarters.
3. Add to a large pan and cover with water. Boil for approximately 15 minutes until soft.
4. Drain and transfer to the roasting tray. Add the garlic powder, onion powder, mixed herbs, salt and pepper. Toss around until well coated and the potatoes are bashed slightly (to help them crisp up more) and then arrange them so that the cut sides are facing down.
5. Roast for 30-40 minutes until crispy and golden.
6. Serve with some torn fresh parsley and extra seasoning, if desired.

## NOTES

1. To use instead of parchment paper or silicone mat. The spray is just watered down olive oil and is only 1 calorie per spray.

Chicken Noodle Soup

Stir-Fry Velveted Chicken and Vegetables

Course: Main Course
Cuisine: Chinese
Prep Time: 25 minutes
Cook Time: 30 minutes
Marinate: 30 minutes
Total Time: 55 minutes
Servings: 4
Calories: 315 kcal

Ingredients
Velveted Chicken
• 1 pound boneless skinless chicken breast
• 1/2 teaspoon salt
• 1 tablespoon rice wine
• 1 large egg white
• 1 tablespoon cornstarch
• 2 tablespoons oil

Vegetables
• 3 cups chicken broth or water
• 1 carrot peeled, cut into 1/2" thick slices
• 4 shitake mushrooms stems removed, quartered
• 1 medium zucchini peeled, seeds scooped out, sliced into 1/2" thick slices
• 1 bunch asparagus tips

Stir-Fry Sauce
- 1 tablespoon soy sauce
- 1 tablespoon oyster sauce
- 1 tablespoon rice wine
- 1/2 teaspoon sugar
- 2 teaspoons cornstarch dissolved in 2 tablespoons cold water
- 2 teaspoons sesame oil

Stir-Fry
- 2 teaspoons oil
- 1 slice ginger peeled, finely minced
- 1/4 cup low sodium chicken stock

Instructions
Velveting Chicken
1. Cut chicken into thin slices, small cubes, or thin strips. Place in bowl and add salt and rice wine; mix well. Whisk egg white with fork until gel is broken down. Add to chicken, along with cornstarch; mix well. Add 1 tablespoons of oil and stir until well mixed. Cover and refrigerate for at least 30 minutes
2. Bring 1 quart of water to a boil. Add 1 tablespoon oil and reduce heat to low. Transfer chicken into pot and stir to separate pieces. Continue to stir until coating turns white. Then immediately strain in colander.
Cooking Vegetables
1. Bring chicken broth to a boil in a saucepan. Add carrot slices. Cook until tender. Remove from pan with slotted

spoon. Add mushrooms and zucchini to chicken broth and cook until tender. Remove from pan with slotted spoon. Add asparagus tips to pan and cook until tender. Remove from pan with slotted spoon. Reserve 1/4 chicken broth stir-fry; store remaining broth for another use.

Stir-Fry Sauce
1. In a small bowl, mix together Stir-Fry Sauce ingredients.
Stir-Frying Chicken and Vegetables
1. Heat oil in a wok or large skillet. Add ginger and stir-fry briefly until fragrant. Add cooked vegetables to wok. Place velveted chicken on top. Add 1/4 cup chicken stock to wok and cover. Cook on high for 1 minute.
2. Add Stir-Fry Sauce and toss well for 1 minute to coat chicken and vegetables with sauce. Serve


## THE GUT REST AND REPAIR SOUP

INGREDIENTS
• 2 cooked chicken breasts-leftovers are ideal for this recipe, or if you're vegan, omit and replace with tofu
• 2 sweet potatoes
• 2 carrots
• 2 medium potatoes
• 750 ml of bone broth or chicken stock
• 1/2 cup of almond milk, this isn't essential, it just gives a creamier taste
• 2 teaspoons of turmeric

• Sprinkle of black pepper

• 1 small piece of ginger

INSTRUCTIONS

1. Peel and slice carrots, sweet potatoes and potatoes; cutting into small chunks.

2. Ensure cooked chicken is chopped finely.

3. Peel ginger and dice finely

WITHOUT A SOUP-MAKER

1. In a large saucepan, add the 750ml of bone broth and 1/2 of the almond milk.

2. Add in the cooked chicken slices (if you've forgotten to cook it, roast the breast for 35 minutes in the oven whilst soup is cooking)

3. Stir in all of the peeled and chopped vegetables, ginger and turmeric.

4. Bring mixture to the boil and then cook on simmer for 35-40 minutes.

5. By this time the vegetables should have soften considerably.

6. You can now use a hand blender or even your nutribullet/blender to blend the mixture into a smooth soup.

7. Add other half of the almond milk to the mixture and stir through.

IF YOU ARE USING A SOUP-MAKER

1. Cook chicken separately-either using leftovers or roast your breast at 200 degrees for around 35 minutes.

2. Add the vegetables, broth, turmeric, ginger and 1/2 the almond milk to the soup maker and set desired program.
3. Once soup is prepared, add in the chicken and the other half of the almond milk.


High-fibre muesli

Ingredients
• 300g jumbo oats
• 100g All-Bran
• 25g wheatgerm
• 100g dark raisins
• 140g ready-to-eat apricots, snipped into chunks
• 50g golden linseed

Method
• Mix everything in a large bowl. You can store this for up to 2 months in an airtight container. When you're ready to serve, pour lots of chilled milk over and let it soak for a few minutes.


Super Easy Low Residue Sweet Potato Hash Browns

Ingredients for my super simple Crohn's recipe: sweet potato hash browns
• 2 sweet potatoes
• 1 tbsp gluten-free flour (or the regular kind if you prefer)

• 2 eggs
• 2 tbsp olive oil

Directions for super simple sweet potato hash browns
1. First up, wash and peel sweet potatoes.
2. Use a grater to grate the sweet potatoes in a mixing bowl to create shredded sweet potato.
3. Use a kitchen roll or a cloth to squeeze the sweet potato to get rid of any extra water. This is important to stop them from being soggy or wet when frying!
4. Place your roll/cloth over the mix, press down hard, and squeeze! Keep doing this until the mix is dry and you think you've gotten rid of all the water.
5. Once that's done, break eggs into the bowl and then add a tablespoon of flour.
6. Mix and coat the sweet potatoes well with the egg and flour.
7. In your frying pan, add olive oil and heat.
8. Use your hands to squash your sweet potato into patty-like shapes.
9. Fry each patty for around 5 minutes until golden brown, then serve.

Ingredients
1. 1tbsp olive oil, coconut oil or ghee
2. 2 tablespoons minced ginger optional
3. 1-2 cloves garlic, minced -optional
4. 175g jasmine rice
5. 1600ml vegetable or chicken stock

6. 1 tsp sea salt

7. Tamari soy sauce for flavouring

8. Chopped chives for topping

9. Optional add ins – cooked shittake mushrooms, cooked plain chicken, handful of soaked sea vegetables

Instructions

1. Rinse the rice with 2 changes of water. Drain and set aside.

2. Heat the oil in a large saucepan. Once hot, add the ginger and garlic and cook for 30 seconds, until they start to become fragrant. Add the drained rice, and sauté for another minute.

3. Carefully pour the broth. Sprinkle in the salt and stir. Bring the broth to a boil, uncovered. Then, turn the heat to a very low heat and cover. Let it simmer for 1 hour – do not take off the lid.

4. Turn off the heat and leave to sit for 15 minutes.

5. Serve the congee in bowls. Top with a little tamari soy sauce, chopped chives if wished.


RAW APPLE CARROT CAKE

Ingredients

1. 2 carrots, grated

2. 2 apples, grated

3. 115g pecans, finely ground

4. 85g desiccated coconut

5. 2tbsp lucuma powder
6. 2tbsp raw cacao powder
7. ½ tsp ground cinnamon
8. Pinch of salt
9. 150g raisins
10. 60g dried apple, soaked for 15 minutes
11. 60g dates, soaked for 15 minutes
12. 1 whole orange, peeled

Instructions
1. Finely grate the apple and carrots. Place in a large bowl with the nuts, lucuma, cacao, cinnamon, salt and raisins.
2. Drain the dried apple and dates and place in a blender with the orange. Process to form a paste. Add to the nut mixture and combined thoroughly. Place the mixture in batches in a food processor and pulse to form a wet dough. Do not over mix.
3. Press the mixture into a greased, lined 20cm (8inch) cake tin and chill for 2-3 hours before serving.

Low-Carb & Keto Greek Chicken Bowls

Prep Time: 15 minutes
Cook Time: 10 minutes
Total Time: 30 minutes
Servings: 4
Course: Main

Cuisine: Greek

Ingredients
Greek Chicken
• 1 lb. chicken breast boneless, skinless, cut into 1-inch (2.5-cm) cubes (455 g)
• 3 tablespoons olive oil (45 ml)
• 2 tablespoons lemon juice
• 1 tablespoon red wine vinegar
• 1 tablespoon Greek seasoning (see notes below)
• 1/4 teaspoon sea salt
Tzatziki sauce
• 8 oz. Greek yoghurt plain, full-fat (224 g)
• 1/2 medium Persian cucumber grated
• 2 cloves garlic grated
• Zest of 1 medium lemon
• 1 tablespoon fresh lemon juice
• 2 tablespoons fresh dill minced
• Sea salt as needed
• Black pepper as needed
Red Wine Vinegar Dressing
• 3 tablespoons olive oil (45 ml)
• 1 tablespoons red wine vinegar
• 1 teaspoon fresh oregano minced
• Sea salt to taste
Salad Toppings
• 1 large Persian cucumber diced
• 1 cup cherry tomatoes halved
• 1/2 cup red onion thinly sliced

• 1/3 cup Kalamata olives pitted
• 4 oz. feta cheese crumbled

Instructions
• To make the chicken, combine the chicken, oil, lemon juice, vinegar, Greek seasoning, and salt in a sealable container. Marinate the chicken in the refrigerator for 30 minutes or up to overnight.
• To make the tzatziki, stir together the yoghurt, cucumber, garlic, lemon zest, lemon juice, dill, salt, and black pepper in a medium bowl. Refrigerate the tzatziki until you are ready to serve.
• Heat a 10-inch (25-cm) or larger cast-iron skillet over medium-high heat. Add the chicken and marinade to the skillet. Cook the chicken for 3 to 4 minutes per side, until it is brown and its internal temperature reaches 165°F (74°C).
• To make the red wine vinegar dressing, whisk together the oil, vinegar, oregano, and salt in a small bowl.
• To assemble the bowls, divide the chicken among four individual serving bowls. Top the chicken with the cucumber, tomatoes, onion, olives, and feta cheese. Pour the red wine vinegar dressing over the bowls and top each bowl with the tzatziki just before serving.

Healthy Chicken Fajitas Meal Prep

PREP TIME: 20 minutes
COOK TIME: 40 minutes
MARINATING: 30 minutes
TOTAL TIME: 1 hour
COURSE/ Meal Prep
SERVINGS: 6 meals
CALORIES: 455 kcal


INGREDIENTS
For The Fajita Chicken:
• ⅓ cup lime juice, (approx. 2-3 limes)
• ¼ cup pineapple juice, no sugar added
• 2 tablespoon low sodium soy sauce
• 1 clove garlic, minced
• 1 tsp. ground cumin
• 1 tsp. paprika
• ½ tsp. red pepper flakes
• 1 tsp. sea salt
• ½ tsp. ground black pepper
• ¼ cup cilantro chopped
• 2 tbsp. olive oil
• 4 6-8 oz. boneless, skinless chicken breasts
For the Fajita Bell Peppers:
• 1 white onion, thinly sliced
• 1 poblano chile, thinly sliced
• 2 red bell peppers, thinly sliced

- 1 green bell pepper, thinly sliced
- 1 tsp. sea salt
- ½ tsp. ground black pepper
- ¼ teaspoon garlic powder

For the Lime & Cilantro Black Beans:
- 1 tablespoon olive oil
- 3 cloves garlic, minced
- ½ jalapeño, (1 tbsp) seeded and finely diced
- ½ teaspoon cumin
- 2 15-ounce cans low sodium black beans, rinsed and drained
- 1 cup low-sodium chicken broth
- 2 tablespoon fresh lime juice
- 2 tablespoon fresh cilantro, chopped
- 1 tsp. sea salt

## INSTRUCTIONS

To Make The Fajita Chicken:
- In a large bowl or ziplock bag, combine the chicken breast with freshly squeezed lime juice, no sugar added pineapple juice, low sodium soy sauce, olive oil, minced garlic, ground cumin, smoked paprika, red pepper flakes, sea salt, ground black pepper, and chopped fresh cilantro.
- Place in the fridge for a minimum of 30 minutes, up to 8 hours.
- Once the chicken is marinated, heat 1 tbsp. olive oil over medium-high heat in a large skillet until hot.

• Add the marinated chicken, cooking on both sides until cooked through, about 4-6 minutes per side.

• Remove the chicken from the pan and set aside to rest. Slice into thin slices.

To Make the Fajita Bell Peppers:

• In the same pan used to cook the chicken, add sliced white onion, sliced poblano pepper, sliced red bell peppers, sliced green bell pepper, sea salt, and ground black pepper, and toss to combine.

• Cook over medium-high heat until the bell peppers and onion are tender, about 4-6 minutes.


To Make the Black Beans:

• Heat oil in large saucepan over medium-high heat.

• Add garlic, jalapeño, and cumin and cook for 1 minute, or until garlic is fragrant.

• Add the beans and broth and cook 5 minutes, stirring occasionally.

• Coarsely mash beans with a potato masher.

• Continue to cook at a simmer for about 8-10 minutes until the mixture is thick, stirring frequently.

• Add in lime juice, cilantro, and sea salt, to taste.

• To assemble the chicken fajita meal prep, start by adding the cilantro lime black beans to your meal prep container, followed by the sliced fajita chicken, and the bell pepper and onion mixture.

Low Calorie Pasta

SERVINGS: 4
PREP: 5 minutes
COOK: 30 minutes
TOTAL: 35 minutes

Ingredients
FOR THE PASTA
• 3 cups low calorie pasta cooked
• 1 cup cottage cheese fat free
• 2 cups fat free mozzarella cheese divided
• 1 large egg
• 1 tablespoon Italian seasonings
FOR THE LOW CALORIE PASTA SAUCE
• 1 1/2 cups tomato sauce passata
• 1 teaspoon Italian seasonings
• 1/2 teaspoon salt
• 1/2 teaspoon pepper
• 1 teaspoon brown sugar substitute

Instructions
• Preheat the oven to 180C/350F. Grease an 8x8-inch baking dish and set aside.
• Cook the low calorie pasta as per the instructions and measure out 3 cups of the cooked noodles. In a separate bowl, whisk the sauce ingredients until combined.

• In a large bowl, mix together half of the pasta sauce, the cottage cheese, one cup of the mozzarella cheese, egg, and Italian herbs. Add the cooked pasta and mix well.

• Spread ¼ cup of the pasta sauce. Add the pasta mixture and then spread the remaining sauce on top. Sprinkle with the remaining mozzarella cheese.

• Cover the baking dish and bake for 35-40 minutes. Uncover and bake until the cheese is melted and bubbling around the sides.


Low Calorie Chicken and Veggies Stir Fry

PREP TIME: 15 minutes
COOK TIME: 15 minutes
TOTAL TIME: 22 minutes
COURSE: Main Course
SERVINGS: 4
CALORIES: 264 Kcal

INGREDIENTS
Ingredients for Stir Fry:
• 2 cups broccoli florets cut in half, see shopping tips
• 2 cups onion diced
• 1 cup carrots diced
• 5 cups cabbage shredded
• 2 cups Chinese pea pods (snow peas) sliced in half
• 1¾ cups cooked chicken breast diced
• cooking spray

• 1 tbsp vegetable, canola, or olive oil
• 3 tbsp water for stir frying
Ingredients for Sauce:
• ⅓ cup plus reduced-sodium soy sauce (for gluten free, use Tamari soy sauce)
• 2 tbsp brown sugar
• 2 tbsp rice vinegar
• 3 tbsp water
• 2 cloves garlic minced
• 2 tsp ginger (from a jar), see shopping tips
• Fresh ground black pepper to taste

## INSTRUCTIONS
• First, prep all vegetables and dice the chicken. Set aside.
• In a small bowl, add all sauce ingredients and mix until well blended. Set aside.
• Coat a large nonstick wok or pan with cooking spray. Heat 1 tablespoon of oil in pan. Add broccoli, onions and carrots and water. Saute over medium-high heat for 5-7 minutes until broccoli is soft.  Add cabbage and chicken. Saute another 3-4 minutes until soft. Turn down to medium heat, stir in pea pods and sauce mixture.  Stir fry for about 2 minutes until all heated through. Stir constantly to blend everything.
• Store any leftovers in the fridge for a few days.

Baked Mediterranean Chicken Thighs

Serving: Main 4 servings
Ready in: 45 mins
Skill level: Easy
Serve with: Your favorite side

Ingredients you'll need
(makes 4 servings)
• 8 chicken thighs, bone-in, skin and excess fat removed
• 1 onion, thinly sliced
• 1 ripe tomato, skin removed and grated
• 2-3 tablespoons of Extra Virgin Olive Oil
• 1 lemon
• 2 sprigs of fresh rosemary (optional)
• 5 garlic cloves, minced
• 1 teaspoon of oregano
• 1 teaspoon of Spanish La Vera smoked paprika
• 1 teaspoon of cumin
• 1 teaspoon of onion powder
• ½ teaspoon of white pepper
• Salt (to taste)

Equipment needed
• 1 baking tray or 12×8 inches Ceramic Baking dish with deep sides (around 2-inches/5 cm)
• Oven

How to make baked Mediterranean chicken thighs

Step 1–Make marinade
• Preheat oven to 200°C / 400°F
• Grate the tomato directly into the baking dish, and add the lemon juice, smoked paprika, oregano, cumin, onion powder, and white pepper. Mix well, add the olive oil and crushed garlic, and mix until the marinade has an even consistency.
Step 2–Add chicken and bake
• Add skinless chicken thighs to the marinade. Add sliced onion between chicken pieces. Season with salt to taste and sprinkle a few sprigs of fresh rosemary on top.
• Bake for 40 minutes.
Step 3–Serve
• Allow to cool for 5 minutes before serving.
• Serve with a squeeze of fresh lemon and some chopped parsley or coriander.


Easy Cajun Shrimp Recipe

Ingredients
• 2 tbsp olive oil
• 1 lb large shrimp, peeled and deveined
• Kosher salt and ground pepper, to taste
• 2 tbsp Cajun seasoning
• Lime wedges, to serve
• For garnish: fresh parsley, finely chopped

• Optional: cooked jasmine rice

Instructions
• Heat the oil in a large skillet over medium-high heat.
• To a large bowl, add the shrimp, salt, pepper, and Cajun seasoning. Toss well to evenly coat.
• Cook for 2-3 minutes per side, or until pink and opaque.
• Garnish with fresh parsley and serve with lime wedges. Serve over cooked rice, if desired.

Notes
• Serving size: half the amount of the shrimp, about half a pound.
• This recipe can easily be doubled to serve 4
• Nutrition facts do not include the rice.
• Use any oil of choice
• You may use lemons if you don't have lime.
• We prefer that you use raw shrimp instead of pre-cooked
• Serve over rice, cauliflower rice, or quinoa


High Fibre Recipe: Saag with Chickpeas

• Prep time: 10 mins
• Cook time: 20 mins
• Servings: 2

Ingredients
• 1 tbsp olive oil

- 1 tsp ginger, grated
- 3 cloves garlic, minced
- 1 onion, diced
- 2 tomatoes, diced
- ½ tsp ground turmeric
- 1 tsp chilli flakes
- 1 tsp ground cumin
- ½ tsp ground coriander
- salt to taste
- 125ml water
- 1 x 400g tin chickpeas, drained
- 250g spinach, roughly chopped
- 1 tsp garam masala
- ½ lemon, juice
- 2 tbsp dried fenugreek leaves, (Kasoori meth)

Instructions

• Heat oil in a pan, add onion, ginger, garlic and sauté until translucent.

• Add tomatoes, turmeric, chilli flakes, cumin, coriander, salt and stir to combine.

• Cook for 4-5 minutes until the tomatoes are soft.

• Add water, chickpeas and continue to cook for another 5-7 minutes. Taste and season with salt as needed.

• Now add the spinach and stir to combine.

• Cook for 4-5 minutes and turn the flame off.

• Finally add garam masala, lemon juice, fenugreek leaves (kasoori methi) and stir together.

• Enjoy as is, or serve with brown rice, quinoa or wholemeal roti on a non-fasting day.


Healthy French Toast

Course: Breakfast
Prep: 2 minutes
Cook: 4 minutes
Total: 6 minutes
Servings: 2 servings
Calories: 315kcal


Ingredients
• 4 slice Whole wheat bread
• 2 Eggs
• 200 ml (0.75 cups) Skimmed milk
• 0.5 teaspoon Cinnamon
• 0.5 teaspoon Ground nutmeg
• 1 tablespoon Maple syrup
• 0.5 teaspoon Vanilla extract
• 0.5 Orange - juice and zest only
• 0.5 tablespoon Butter

Instructions
• Add 2 Eggs, 200 ml Skimmed milk, 0.5 teaspoon Cinnamon, 0.5 teaspoon Ground nutmeg, 0.5 teaspoon Vanilla extract, 1 tablespoon Maple syrup and the juice and zest of 0.5 Orange to a bowl and mix well.

• Dip 4 slices Whole wheat bread into the mixture one slice at a time until the mixture soaks into it.
• Add 0.5 tablespoon Butter to a pan and add the soaked slices of bread. Cook for around 2-3 minutes on each side, turned every minute or so.

Recipe tips
• To freeze, allow to cool to room temperature and then individually wrap and then store in a freezer bag. Once defrosted you can reheat in the toaster.
• Try to use 2 day old bread, as this will stop the French toast from becoming too soggy.
• Make a toddler friendly version of this by leaving out the maple syrup and then cutting it in to sticks.
• You can lighten this up even more by using just egg whites, rather than whole eggs.


## THE ULTIMATE LOW-CARB STIR-FRY

COOK TIME: 10 MINUTES
TOTAL TIME: 10 MINUTES
SERVINGS: 2 PEOPLE

INGREDIENTS
• 1 Tbsp avocado oil
• 1 lbs ground chicken - (or turkey or shrimps)
• 2-3 cloves crushed garlic

- 1 Tbsp peeled and grated ginger
- 1 bag Mann's Rainbow Salad
- 1/4 cup soy sauce - (Tamari for Gluten-Free)
- 4 sliced scallions
- 1 Tbsp sesame seed oil

INSTRUCTIONS
- Add avocado oil to a hot pan.
- Add ground chicken to pan and break up with a wooden spoon and stir-fry until almost cooked through.
- Stir in ginger and garlic.
- Add Mann's Rainbow Salad vegetables and soy sauce and stir-fry until vegetables reach desired consistency. 2-5 minutes.
- Sprinkle sliced scallions and drizzle sesame seed oil over everything, give it one last quick stir and serve immediately.

Healthier Vegan Pistachio Halva

PREP TIME: 10 minutes
CHILL TIME: 1 hour
COURSE: Dessert
SERVINGS: 10
CALORIES: 175 kcal

INGREDIENTS

- 200 g Medjool dates or any soft dates
- 180 ml tahini
- 1/2 tsp cardamom optional
- Pinch of salt
- 20 g pistachios roughly chopped

INSTRUCTIONS
- Add the dates and tahini to a food processor along with a pinch of salt and cardamom and blend until you have a smooth, well-combined mixture.
- Transfer into moulds, then top with some pistachios and freeze for 1 hour.
- Alternatively you can press down into a loaf tin lined with baking paper, freeze for 1 hour, then slice into squares.
- Store in an air-tight container in the fridge for up to 5 days.

Healthy Chicken Quesadillas

SERVINGS: 4

Ingredients
- 1 cup cooked boneless skinless chicken breast
- 1/2 cup canned diced tomatoes with green chilies
- 1/2 cup canned black beans, rinsed and drained
- 1/2 cup canned corn, rinsed and drained
- 1/4 cup cilantro, chopped
- 1/2 tsp garlic powder

• 1/2 tsp onion powder
• 1/2 tsp cumin
• 1/4 tsp oregano
• 4 flour tortillas
• 1 1/3 cups reduced fat shredded pepper jack cheese (or other cheese)

Instructions

1. Combine the chicken, tomatoes, black beans, corn, cilantro, garlic powder, onion powder, cumin, and oregano. Season with salt and pepper.

2. Heat a nonstick skillet over medium high heat. Place the tortilla in the skillet and sprinkle one half with about 1.5 tbsp of cheese. Spread with about 1/2 cup of the chicken filling. Top with another 1.5 tbsp of cheese. Fold the tortilla over and cook on one side until cheese is melting and the tortilla begins to brown. Flip over and cook on the other side for 2-3 minites more until tortilla browns and cheese it fully melted. Repeat with remaining quesadillas.

3. You can also make full-size quesadillas instead of folding the tortillas in half. Just make sure to note that the serving size would be half a larger quesadilla.


Low Carb Greek Yoghurt Chicken

Prep Time: 10 minutes
Cook Time: 20 minutes
Total Time: 30 minutes

Serving: 4

Ingredients
• oil spray
• 5 oz. plain greek yogurt, (I used 5% fat yogurt)
• 2 tablespoon mayonnaise
• ½ cup grated parmesan cheese
• 1 teaspoon garlic powder
• 1 teaspoon salt
• ½ teaspoon black pepper
• 1.5 lb. chicken tenders (whole) or chicken breasts (cut in quarters)
• Parsley, (chopped, for garnish)

Instructions
• Preheat oven to 375°F. Lightly coat a 12 inch oven proof pan or 9×9 baking dish with nonstick oil spray and set aside.
• In a medium bowl, mix together the greek yogurt, mayonnaise, Parmesan cheese, garlic powder, salt and pepper.
• Add chicken into the bowl with yogurt mixture and coat the mixture all over the chicken.
• Move chicken to a baking dish (or oven proof pan). Chicken should be thinly coated with the yogurt mixture. Don't put too much or any additional mixture leftover.
• Bake for 25-30 minutes, or until the chicken is cooked through.

• Turn the oven to broil and place the pan under the broiler for 2-3 minutes until lightly browned on top.
• Optional: garnish with chopped parsley.

High Protein Chicken Alfredo

Cooking Method: Blender, Food Processor, Stovetop
Cuisine: Poultry
Prep Time: 20 mins
Cook Time: 10 mins
Total Time: 30 mins
Servings: 4
Calories: 589

Ingredients
• 1 cup Low Fat Cottage Cheese
• 1 1/2 cup Unsweetened Almond Milk
• 2 tbsp Cornstarch
• 1 cup Parmesan Cheese
• 1 tsp Garlic Powder
• 1 tsp Dried Parsley
• 1 tsp Pepper
• 1/2 tsp Nutmeg
• 1 Box of Banza Pasta
• 600 g Broccoli
• 12 oz Chicken Breasts

Instructions

• First, cook your pasta according to the box.

• For your broccoli, you can use fresh or frozen. I use frozen broccoli that I warmed in a pan. You can also steam.

• Next, cook your chicken to your liking. Another option would also be to buy pre-made chicken.

• Divide all your ingredients into four meal prep containers - 4oz of chicken, 150g of broccoli, 1/2 cup of alfredo sauce and 2 oz of dried pasta.

Alfredo Sauce

• In a blender or food processor, combine your cottage cheese, milk, cornstarch, parmesan cheese, garlic, parsley, pepper and nutmeg. Blend until smooth and set aside.

• Add your Alfredo sauce to a sauce pan and cook on low medium for 3 to 5 minutes until thickened.


## MEDITERRANEAN ROASTED VEGETABLES

PREP TIME: 10 minutes
COOK TIME: 20 minutes
TOTAL TIME: 30
COURSE: Side Dish
CUISINE: Mediterranean
SERVINGS: 10
CALORIES: 66 kcal

INGREDIENTS
• 1 pint Tomatoes

- 1 Red Onion
- 2 Orange Bell Peppers
- 1 medium Zucchini
- 1 medium Yellow Squash
- 3 Tablespoons Olive Oil
- 1 Tablespoon Fresh Thyme
- 1 teaspoon Oregano
- 1 teaspoon Garlic Powder
- ½ teaspoon Cumin
- Black Pepper to taste

INSTRUCTIONS

- Cut the vegetables into similar sized pieces, and then toss them together in a large mixing bowl with the olive oil, spices, and fresh thyme.
- Spread the vegetables into a single layer on a baking sheet. You may need two baking sheets depending on their size.
- Roast at 425 degrees on the middle rack of your oven for 20 minutes.

NOTES

- I chose to use a rainbow of veggies: tomato, orange bell peppers, yellow squash, zucchini, and red onion. Feel free to swap these out with some of YOUR favorites, such as mushrooms, carrot, fennel, or eggplant.
- You can substitute 1 teaspoon dried thyme for the fresh thyme.

• Leftover vegetables can be stored in an airtight container in your refrigerator for up to 3 days.

The Best Keto Cheese Sauce

Ingredients (makes about 1 cup, 4 servings)
• 1/4 cup heavy whipping cream (60 ml/ 2 fl oz)
• 2 tbsp unsalted butter (28 g/ 1 oz)
• 1/4 cup cream cheese or soft goat cheese (60 g/ 2.1 oz)
• 1/2 cup grated cheddar or hard cheese of choice (60 g/ 2.1 oz)
• pinch of sea salt, if needed
• 2 tbsp water or more cream if you need to thin it down

Instructions
1. Place the cream and butter into a small sauce pan and gently heat up. Add the grated cheddar cheese (or any hard cheese of choice) and cream cheese.
2. Stir until melted and bring to a simmer. Once you see bubbles, take off the heat.
3. Mix until smooth and creamy. If you prefer a thicker sauce, cook for 3-5 more minutes while stirring. If too thick, add a splash of water or cream.
4. Serve immediately with steamed vegetables, fish and meat. The cooled sauce can also be stored in the fridge in a sealed jar for up to 5 days.

Weight-Loss Cabbage Soup

Active Time: 35 mins
Total Time: 55 mins
Servings: 6
Yield: 12 cups

Ingredients
• 2 tablespoons extra-virgin olive oil
• 1 medium onion, chopped
• 2 medium carrots, chopped
• 2 stalks celery, chopped
• 1 medium red bell pepper, chopped
• 2 cloves garlic, minced
• 1 ½ teaspoons Italian seasoning
• ½ teaspoon ground pepper
• ¼ teaspoon salt
• 8 cups low-sodium vegetable broth
• 1 medium head green cabbage, halved and sliced
• 1 large tomato, chopped
• 2 teaspoons white-wine vinegar

Directions
1. Heat oil in a large pot over medium heat. Add onion, carrots and celery. Cook, stirring, until the vegetables begin to soften, 6 to 8 minutes. Add bell pepper, garlic, Italian seasoning, pepper and salt and cook, stirring, for 2 minutes.
2. Add broth, cabbage and tomato; increase heat to medium-high and bring to a boil. Reduce heat to maintain a

simmer, partially cover and cook until all the vegetables are tender, 15 to 20 minutes more. Remove from heat and stir in vinegar.

## LOW CARB TORTILLAS

Prep Time: 5 minutes
Cook Time: 10 minutes
Chilling Time: 30 minutes
Total Time: 45 minutes
Course: Main Course
Servings: 6
Calories: 231 kcal

## INGREDIENTS
• 1 ½ cup almond flour 150g (reduce by 2 tablespoons if you're using super-fine almond flour)
• ⅔ cup flax meal 80g
• 2 tablespoon whole psyllium husks 8g (or 1 tablespoon psyllium husk powder)
• 1 large egg whisked lightly with a fork
• 10 tablespoon lukewarm water
• ¾ teaspoon sea salt optional

INSTRUCTIONS
• Place all the dry ingredients in a mixing bowl (almond flour, flax meal, psyllium husk and salt). Mix well to combine.

Greek Quinoa Salad

INGREDIENTS
• 1 cup dry quinoa
• 2 cups broth or water
• 1 cup chopped tomatoes
• 1 cup chopped cucumber
• 1 cup chopped bell pepper
• 1/2 cup diced green onion green parts only
• 1 cup feta
• Olives optional
• 2 tablespoons extra virgin olive oil (can use garlic infused oil, see notes)
• 3 tablespoons lemon juice
• 1 tsp basil dried
• 1 tsp oregano dried
• 1/4 tsp salt
• 1/4 tsp pepper

INSTRUCTIONS
• Pour the broth or water into a medium saucepan and bring to a boil. Add the quinoa and reduce heat to low. Simmer

with lid on for 15 minutes until water is absorbed. Pour the quinoa into a large bowl and let cool.

• Wash and dry your vegetables. Chop the veggies and feta into bite sized pieces.

• Mix together the oil, lemon juice, basil, oregano, salt and pepper in a small bowl.

• Once the quinoa is cool, add the vegetables and dressing to the bowl and mix well. Taste and add more seasoning as needed. If you use a salt-free both or water you may want to add more salt.

## GLUTEN-FREE COCONUT CHICKEN CURRY RECIPE (LOW FODMAP + DAIRY FREE)

INGREDIENTS
FOR THE SPICE BLEND:
• 2 tbsp curry powder (ensure it is low FODMAP-see FAQ section above for links)
• 1 tbsp paprika
• 1 tsp cinnamon
• 1/2 tsp ground ginger
• 1/2 tsp asafoetida
FOR THE CURRY:
• 1 tbsp garlic infused olive oil
• 2 chicken breasts chopped
• 200 ml canned coconut milk 180ml if low FODMAP elimination phase

• 200 ml Greek yoghurt lactose-free if low FODMAP, dairy-free coconut yoghurt if dairy-free
• 1 tbsp tomato puree
• 1 tbsp lemon juice optional
• 1-2 handfuls of spinach

TO SERVE:
• Handful of fresh chives chopped
• Fresh coriander
• Basmati rice I add 1 tsp of turmeric to mine to make it yellow

INSTRUCTIONS
• Place your pan over a medium heat and add a tbsp of garlic-infused oil. Once heated, add your chicken chunks and fry until almost sealed.
• Add your spice mix and stir fry for 1 minute.
• Next add your coconut milk and tomato puree. Stir and then simmer for about 10-15 minutes.
• Add your spinach and lemon juice, if using. Cook until the spinach has wilted down.
• Lastly, add your yoghurt and mix in.
• Sprinkle of some fresh chives and top with fresh coriander! Serve up with basmati rice and my 3-ingredient gluten-free naan bread.

NOTES
1. A safe serving size for the elimination phase of the low FODMAP diet is third of this entire recipe.

# Low Fiber Smoothie Recipes

Prune Smoothie

Ingredients
• 1 cup ice
• 1/2 cup unsweetened almond milk
• 1/2 cup water
• 1/2 frozen banana
• 1 cup baby spinach or other greens
• 1/4 cup prunes
• 1/2 tablespoon chia seeds
• 1 tablespoon honey or maple syrup

Instructions
• Put all ingredients into a blender and pulse/puree until smooth.


Green Protein Smoothie

Ingredients
• 1 frozen banana
• 1 scoop vanilla protein powder
• 1 cup cold unsweetened vanilla almond milk, or other milk
• 2 cups baby spinach, loosely packed
• 1 Tablespoon chia seeds

Instructions
• Place all ingredients into a high-powered blender and blend until smooth



High Protein Vegan Peanut Butter Strawberry Banana Smoothie

Prep Time: 3 minutes
Cook Time: 0 minutes
Total Time: 3 minutes

Ingredients
• 1 banana, ripe (frozen preferred)
• 1 cup frozen strawberries
• ¼ cup old fashioned oats
• 2 tablespoon hemp seeds
• 2 tablespoon peanut butter
• 1 tablespoon ground flaxseed
• 1 cup non-dairy unsweetened milk
• 1-2 dates, pitted

Instructions
• Add all the ingredients to a high powered blender.  If using fresh strawberries or banana, you may want to add ice to make it cold.
• Blend until smooth, scraping down the sides if needed.
Chocolate Peanut Butter High-Fiber Smoothie

Ingredients
- 12–16 ounces of filtered water (about 2 cups)
- 1 frozen banana
- 2 teaspoons raw cacao
- 1 tablespoon unsweetened organic peanut butter
- 1 teaspoon raw honey (local if possible)
- 2 teaspoons hemp seeds (aka hemp hearts)
- 1 tablespoon psyllium husk fiber
- a few drops of high-quality vanilla extract
- 2–3 ice cubes
- Optional: 1 serving of chocolate or vanilla high-quality protein powder for extra protein

Instructions
1. Blend all ingredients on high in a high-speed blender. Drink right away, or let sit in the refrigerator for 30 minutes to thicken if you want to eat it with a spoon.
2. Optional: Sprinkle the top with hemp seeds for a pretty garnish.


Mango Spinach Smoothie (with Protein)

Equipment
- Blender
- Chef's Knife
- Cutting Board

Ingredients
• 1 cup mango chunks fresh or frozen
• ½ cup frozen banana
• 2 cup baby spinach loosely packed
• 1 cup water or coconut water, juice, or milk of choice
• Juice of 1 lemon or 1-2 tablespoons of lemon juice
• 2 scoops vanilla protein powder (or ½ cup Greek yogurt)

Instructions
• Add all of your ingredients to a blender.
• Cover and blend until smooth. Sweeten to taste with honey if you like.

Notes
1. Optional add-ins: 1 tablespoon honey (or maple syrup or agave)1 tablespoon chia seeds (or ground flax seed)
2. Nutrition information calculated using vanilla protein powder and water, and without any of the optional add-ins listed above.
3. For a vegan smoothie: This smoothie is naturally dairy free and gluten free, but be sure to use a plant based protein powder for a vegan version.
4. For a paleo smoothie: This smoothie is naturally dairy free and grain free, but be sure to use a paleo friendly protein powder for a paleo compliant version.
5. For more ingredient swaps, modifications, tip & tricks (like how to make this into a smoothie bowl!) see the full blog post above.

Superfood Green Smoothie

Ingredients
• ½ avocado, peeled & pitted
• 1 banana
• ½ cup spinach
• ½ cup ice cubes
• 1 cup almond milk
• 1 tbsp vegan protein powder, clink link for the one I recommend
• 1 tbsp flaxseed
• 1 tsp honey
• ¼ tsp ground cinnamon

Instructions
• Add the avocado, banana, spinach, ice cubes and almond milk to a blender.
• Add the protein powder, flax seed, honey and ground cinnamon.
• Blend until smooth and creamy.
Notes
• Vegan: to make this recipe vegan, substitute agave nectar, coconut nectar or maple syrup for the honey.

## FRUIT AND OATMEAL SMOOTHIE

## INGREDIENTS
• 1 cup ice
• 1 cup mixed berries

- 1/2 cup oats
- 1 cup almond milk
- 1/2 cup Greek yogurt (plain & low fat)
- 2 tablespoons flaxseed meal

INSTRUCTIONS
- Add the ice and fruit to a food processor or blender.
- Blend together until ice is crushed
- Next, add the oats and flaxseed meal to the food processor and blend until the oats are incorporated fully.
- Add the yogurt and milk and pulse a few more times until creamy.

Low Carb Raspberry Smoothie

Prep: 5 minutes
Cook: 0 minutes
Total: 5 minutes
Servings: 2 people

Ingredients
- 1 medium avocado peeled and pitted
- 3/4 cup raspberry
- 1 tbsp lemon juice
- 1 ½ cup unsweetened coconut milk
- 1 scoop of sugar-free vanilla protein powder

Instructions

• Add all the ingredients to a blender.
• Puree for about 30 seconds.
• Taste to adjust flavor and serve immediately.

Tips
• You can use fresh or frozen raspberries for this raspberry smoothie recipe.
• For a thicker smoothie, you can add ice to the blender.
• Feel free to swap the coconut milk or almond milk.
• To store: You can store the raspberry smoothie for a day in the fridge but you'll have to give it a mix as the ingredients may separate.

Fruit smoothie breakfast bowl recipe

Ingredients
• 300g natural yogurt
• 2 bananas (super-ripe)
• 1 pinch cinnamon
• 30g rolled oats
• 120g frozen mixed berries
• Milk (optional)
• 1 handful of shredded wheat bitesize cereal (or other low-sugar cereal, such as Weetabix, or no-added-sugar muesli)
• 2 tbsp peanut butter
• 2 tbsp 4 seed mix (or mixed nuts)
• Fresh seasonal fruit, such as raspberries, to serve (optional)

Method

• Put the yogurt, bananas, cinnamon and oats in a blender and blitz until smooth. Pour out around two-thirds of the mixture and divide between your bowls, glasses or lolly moulds.

• Add the frozen berries to the blender, reserving a few for the topping, and blitz again until smooth, adding a splash of milk to loosen, if needed.

• Divide the berry mixture between your bowls, glasses or lolly moulds, then swirl the two together to create a rippled effect.

• Serve with a mixture of toppings: a sprinkling of cereal, a dollop of peanut butter, a scattering of nuts and seeds, and some fresh fruit. Delicious.


Berry High Fiber Smoothie

Prep Time: 5 minutes
Total Time: 5 minutes

Ingredients
• 1 cup milk of choice
• ¾ cup plain Greek yogurt
• 1 cup frozen raspberries
• 1 cup frozen blueberries
• 1 banana frozen
• 2 tablespoon flax seeds
• ½ an avocado peeled and pit removed

• ½ cup white navy beans rinsed and drained
Optional:
• 2 tablespoon vanilla protein powder
• Top with additional berries and fresh mint if desired

Instructions
• In a high powered blender start by adding milk and Greek yogurt. Add remaining ingredients and blend until smooth.
• Pour into two glasses and enjoy!

Notes
1. I have included an estimation of the nutrition information for this recipe below. However, always remember a recipe is so much more than just nutritional content and these numbers do not need to dictate your food choices. Please don't forget that both your body and soul need nourishment! The owner of this website is not liable for this estimation.

Smoothie bowl

Ingredients
• 200g frozen mixed berries
• 1 ripe banana
• 75ml oat milk
• 1 tsp maple syrup
• ½ tbsp vanilla protein powder, vegan version if needed

To top
• Sliced kiwis, bananas and fresh berries
• 25g granola
• 1 tbsp mixed nuts and seeds
• 1 tbsp almond butter


Method
• Put the berries, banana, oat milk, maple syrup and protein powder in a powerful blender and blend until smooth. Add a splash more milk if needed, but remember it needs to be quite thick.
• Spoon the smoothie into a bowl and dot over the fresh fruit, granola and mixed nuts and seeds. Drizzle over the almond butter to serve.


Low Sugar Simple Green Smoothie

Prep Time: 5 minutes
Total Time: 5 minutes
Ingredients
• 2 cups Almond Breeze Unsweetened Vanilla Almondmilk
• ¼-1/2 cup ice cubes (optional)
• ½ frozen banana and/or stevia, to taste
• 1 ½ cups baby spinach, baby kale and/or "power greens" mix
• 1 tablespoon peanut butter or almond butter
• 1 tablespoons ground flax seeds

• 1 tablespoon chia seeds
• Pinch sea salt
• Optional add-ins: spirulina or other "green" powder and/or collagen powder

Instructions
• In a blender, combine the Almond Breeze Unsweetened Vanilla Almondmilk, ice cubes (if using), banana and/or stevia, greens, nut butter, flax seeds, chia seeds and a pinch of sea salt. If using any add-ins, throw them in. Blend on high until the smoothie is very smooth, 30 seconds - 2 minutes, depending on your blender.
• Pour the smoothie into a glass. Enjoy it right away, or let it sit for up to 1 hour before drinking (the smoothie will thicken as it sits).

Notes
• I prefer to use baby spinach, baby kale and/or a "power greens" mix for this smoothie, which are milder in flavor than mature greens (which will overpower the other flavors).
• Almond Breeze Unsweetened Vanilla Almondmilk gives the smoothie creaminess and a delicious flavor without any added sugar.
• The ice in this recipe is optional (depending on how cold you like your beverages!).
• Using frozen (instead of fresh) banana will create a richer, thicker texture, but if you don't have one you can use fresh banana instead.

• You can use either powdered stevia or liquid stevia, according to what you have and like.
• For more protein, feel free to add a neutral collagen powder.
• A green powder mix gives the smoothie a bigger boost of vitamins and minerals, but it's optional (this is the brand I use).
• A pinch of sea salt balances the flavors and provides electrolytes.

# 7-Day Low-Fiber Diet Meal Plan

Day 1
• Breakfast: Scrambled eggs with white toast and a small serving of low-fat yogurt.
• Lunch: Grilled chicken breast with white rice and steamed carrots.
• Dinner: Baked salmon with mashed potatoes and green beans (well-cooked).
• Snacks: Low-fiber crackers with cream cheese or a small serving of canned peaches.
Day 2
• Breakfast: Low-fiber cereal or cream of rice and a side of scrambled eggs.
• Lunch: Turkey and cheese sandwich on white bread with a side of applesauce.
• Dinner: Tofu stir-fry with white rice and cooked zucchini.
• Snacks: Smoothie made with a ripe banana, low-fat milk, and a scoop of protein powder.
Day 3
• Breakfast: Pancakes made with white flour, topped with maple syrup, and a side of scrambled eggs.
• Lunch: Tuna salad with canned tuna and mayonnaise served on white bread.
• Dinner: Roast chicken with mashed potatoes and cooked spinach.
• Snacks: Low-fiber crackers and cheese with a side of cubed watermelon.
Day 4

• Breakfast: French toast made with white bread, served with a dollop of Greek yogurt and a sprinkle of cinnamon.

• Lunch: Chicken noodle soup made with white pasta and well-cooked chicken pieces, with a side of ripe nectarines.

• Dinner: Baked cod with white rice and steamed green beans.

• Snacks: Rice cakes with a small serving of fruit cocktail (canned in juice).

Day 5

• Breakfast: Smoothie made with banana, low-fat yogurt, and a handful of spinach leaves (strained if necessary).

• Lunch: Grilled cheese sandwich on white bread with a side of tomato soup (strained), and melon slices.

• Dinner: Pork tenderloin with mashed sweet potatoes and cooked carrots.

• Snacks: Low-fiber crackers with cottage cheese or a small serving of canned mandarin oranges.

Day 6

• Breakfast: Scrambled eggs with white toast and a side of sliced banana.

• Lunch: Ham and cheese wrap made with a white tortilla, served with potato salad.

• Dinner: Turkey meatballs with white pasta and cooked asparagus.

• Snacks: Rice pudding.

Day 7

• Breakfast: Breakfast burrito made with scrambled eggs and cheese in a white tortilla.

• Lunch: Creamy chicken and rice soup (strained) with a side of white bread.
• Dinner: Beef pot roast with mashed potatoes and cooked squash.
• Snacks: Low-fiber crackers with cream cheese or a small serving of canned fruit cocktail.

# CONCLUSION

It's a good idea to consult with a doctor or dietitian if you plan on making significant changes to your diet. Before you cut out all potentially hard-to-digest foods, you may find it helpful to keep a food diary or use an app to log your meals.

Record what you've eaten, what time you ate it, and how the food makes you feel. That way, you can identify and avoid foods that cause gas, bloating, stomach pain, or other discomfort.

You can also provide this information to your healthcare professional to help diagnose and treat any underlying medical conditions that may contribute to your symptoms.